banish back pain with Alexander Technique

Richard Craze

For UK order enquiries: please contact Bookpoint Ltd,
130 Milton Park, Abingdon, Oxon OX14 4SB.
Telephone: +44 (0) 1235 827720. *Fax:* +44 (0) 1235 400454.
Lines are open 09.00–17.00, Monday to Saturday, with a 24-hour
message answering service. Details about our titles and how to
order are available at www.hoddereducation.com

British Library Cataloguing in Publication Data: a catalogue record
for this title is available from the British Library.

First published in UK 2011 by Hodder Headline Plc,
338 Euston Road, London NW1 3BH.

Typeset by MPS Limited, a Macmillan Company.

Printed in Great Britain for Hodder Education, an Hachette UK Company,
338 Euston Road, London NW1 3BH, by CPI Cox & Wyman, Reading,
Berkshire RG1 8EX.

The publisher has used its best endeavours to ensure that the URLs
for external websites referred to in this book are correct and active
at the time of going to press. However, the publisher and the
author have no responsibility for the websites and can make no
guarantee that a site will remain live or that the content will remain
relevant, decent or appropriate.

Hachette UK's policy is to use papers that are natural, renewable
and recyclable products and made from wood grown in sustainable
forests. The logging and manufacturing processes are expected to
conform to the environmental regulations of the country of origin.

Impression number   10 9 8 7 6 5 4 3 2 1

Year   2015 2014 2013 2012 2011

Contents

1

a history
of the
Alexander
Technique

To understand the Alexander Technique fully it is essential to know who Frederick Matthias Alexander was, and how and why he developed his Technique. Alexander was a Tasmanian actor who suffered from a recurring problem of voice loss. By watching himself in a mirror as he rehearsed, he was able to identify the cause of the problem, which was threefold: he tensed his neck causing his head to go back; he tightened his throat muscles; and he took a short, deep breath. Alexander discovered how to correct these habits and this led to the development of the Technique. The fundamental principles that he discovered can be summed up as: *the manner of doing* – how we develop the habits that precede movements; *not doing* – the more we try to correct the fault, the worse we can make it, and by not doing we can learn more; *primary control* – the relationship between head, neck and torso influences the entire body; and **inhibiting** – old habits are stronger than the desire to change.

In order to understand the Alexander Technique fully it is essential to know how and why it came about. You may be tempted to skip this chapter, but I would seriously recommend that you don't. Without knowing who Frederick Matthias Alexander was and how he developed his Technique you could miss a lot of vital clues as to how it works.

Most books that concern therapies of one sort or another include case histories, but for the Alexander Technique the best case history is the man himself.

Alexander's early history

Alexander was born into a poor family in Wynyard, Tasmania, in 1869. He was the eldest of eight children and grew up on a remote farm in north-west Tasmania. As a child he was weak and sickly and suffered from continual breathing problems. Today he may well have been diagnosed as asthmatic. At times he was too ill to attend school and was kept at home where he managed to learn whatever he could. Naturally, being at home a lot led to him growing up isolated from other children. From an early age he was individualistic and unorthodox and was labelled at that time as precocious.

From the age of about nine his health began to improve although he continued to stay at home. He began to learn how to manage horses, which his family bred, exercising them and training them. A passion for horses stayed with him throughout his life. He also began to show an interest in the theatre – it seemed a natural path for someone as confident and outgoing as Alexander to follow. Remember it was the 1870s, there was no television, not even radio, and he lived on a farm a long way away from the nearest neighbours, with seven younger brothers and sisters. What could be more natural than for him to become the entertainer for their benefit? Alexander discovered Shakespeare around this time and began to learn how to recite his favourite speeches. He set his heart on a life as an actor but in 1885, when he was still only 16, the family suffered a series of disastrous financial setbacks and Alexander had no choice but to look around for a regular job.

A young man in Melbourne

Alexander had to take whatever was offered and found himself in the mining town of Mount Bischoff (Tasmania) – as a clerk in a tin mine. Somehow he managed to stick at it, sending money home regularly, until three years later when he had managed to save enough to get himself to Melbourne. By now the family's fortunes had revived somewhat and Alexander was able to use his savings to rent board and lodgings in the city and to pay for acting lessons. He also discovered a new passion for music.

He was 19 years old and living in a big city for the first time. He entered into the spirit of his new life completely. He went to the theatre as often as possible, mixed with other actors, visited art galleries, attended concerts, and even managed to organize his own amateur dramatic company.

Casual work

These were exciting times for the young actor. When he ran short of money he took casual jobs as and when he could find them – as a bookkeeper and a clerk, a store assistant and a tea-taster. He never managed to keep any job for very long for three reasons. First, he despised what he called 'trade'; second, he suffered from a short fuse and a fairly violent temper; and third, he couldn't be bothered to dedicate himself to any job for the simple reason that he knew he was going to be an actor – and a good one.

Speechless

As his popularity began to grow and he was called upon more and more to give his one-man show, he began to suffer from a complaint that seemed utterly disastrous for an actor – he lost his voice.

The first few times it happened he was able to rest for a day or two and, when he had recovered his voice, he could continue with his shows. But the problem not only persisted, it actually began to get worse. He tried all the usual remedies of doctors' prescriptions and throat medicine but nothing seemed to work. The more shows he did, the worse his voice got. He went to various voice teachers and doctors and the only cure was complete rest.

He gave up speaking completely, on one doctor's advice, for two weeks. At the end of the fortnight his voice was back to normal and he gave a show that evening. Half-way through the show his voice went completely and he was forced to abandon the performance. The same doctor recommended that this time he give up speaking for a month. Alexander was not impressed. 'Surely,' he asked, 'if my voice was all right at the beginning of the show but let me down half-way through then it must have been something I was doing that caused it to go?' The doctor thought he might well be right but was unable to offer any further help.

The manner of doing

Alexander took to watching himself in a mirror as he rehearsed to see if there was anything he was doing that was causing the voice loss. He knew his ordinary speaking voice was not affected – it was only when he was reciting that the voice loss was triggered. He watched himself in the mirror as he spoke normally and again as he recited. He noticed that while he spoke normally nothing much happened, but that just before he began to recite he did three things: he tensed his neck causing his head to go back, he tightened his throat muscles, and he took a short deep breath. As he recited he noticed that he did these three things constantly, even exaggerating them quite wildly at times as the passion of his acting overtook him. But this was how he had been trained to project his voice as a professional actor. He found that even when he spoke normally he was still doing these three things but on a much smaller scale, he just hadn't been able to see it before.

Alexander was observing what he called his *manner of doing*.

Once he had seen his manner of doing he thought, quite rightly, that if he was able to stop doing the three things then his voice must improve. And he thought it would be easy to stop doing them. But he was wrong. He managed to stop tensing his neck but when he tried to control the tightening of his throat muscles or the sharp intake of breath just before he began to recite, he was unable to break the habit.

Not doing

Unable to correct his habits, he was unable to rectify the problem. He decided that he would take it one step at a time, beginning with the neck tensing because he found he could control this – and this is where he made the discovery that was to lead to the Alexander Technique. He found that if he didn't tense his neck and stopped trying to correct the other two faults they disappeared on their own. By *not doing* he managed to do. He realized that by not doing he was making a conscious choice to do. This is the basic fundamental principle behind all of his subsequent teaching. This choice, he reasoned, was responsible for the quality of his performance. He called this capability of choice *use*.

He wanted to take this discovery further and practised putting his head forwards, as he had observed that by tensing his neck it was pulled backwards. He thought that if he put his head forwards he might improve his voice even more. While doing this he noticed, in his mirrors, that as soon as he put his head forwards he again tightened his throat muscles causing his larynx to constrict, and he also lifted his chest, narrowing his back which made him physically shorter. By merely putting his head forwards he changed his entire body shape and tension.

He realized that this tension throughout his body influenced everything about him. His voice was not the problem, how he stood was not the cause, and trying to correct it all was not the cure. What he had to learn to do was *not* to do. He knew that if he put his head up and forwards he could maintain his acting voice indefinitely. All he had to do was not tense anything. Again he used mirrors to make sure he was doing exactly what he wanted to and this was when he made his second most important discovery. By observing himself he realized that when he *thought* he was putting his head up and forwards he was actually not doing that. He was still pulling it back.

He knew he had to do two things: *prevent* the movement backwards and *do* the movement forwards. But the more he tried, the harder it seemed to become. It was easy in theory but impossible in practice. The more he tried to do, the worse it became. He realized that the head position dominated the entire body attitude – but he couldn't seem to move his head as he wanted to. He also saw that his head was invariably not where he thought it was. He realized that the relationship between head, neck and body influences the entire body posture and position. He called this relationship *primary control*.

Trusting his feelings

He was fascinated by these discoveries and began to apply them to all aspects of his life. He watched himself walking, standing, talking, gesturing and so on. He noticed that all movements were influenced by his head position – when it was unbalanced or wrong then his entire body was tensed badly. However, he couldn't tell when it was right just by feeling or thought. He could see it physically in the mirrors but what he saw as wrong often, if not always, *felt* right. And when it felt wrong to him it looked right in the mirror.

He realized that he had developed certain habits of holding his head in a particular way for so long that it had become an unconscious trait. And this trait or habit felt right *because* he had been doing it for so long. The correct head placement felt wrong because it was new and unaccustomed. It dawned on him that he couldn't trust his feelings about where and how he was holding his body. This quite shocked him and seems, even now, to unsettle some of the basic assumptions we make about our lives. If we can't trust our perceptions of where we are and what we are doing, then what can we trust? Alexander decided that it must be possible to restore the trust. If *doing* was wrong then he would have to look more closely at *not doing*.

Inhibition

As he watched and tried to change he made another important discovery: the habit was always stronger than the desire to change. It seemed as though he only had to think about doing something before all the old habits kicked in automatically and he would tense something somewhere that he didn't want to tense.

Putting it all together

Alexander began to put all the discoveries together. He practised at first just reciting one sentence and, as he did so, bringing into play the things he had learnt from observation:

1 Inhibiting the immediate response to speak and thus stopping the habits at source.
2 Consciously projecting the primary control directions for the improved 'use of self' which were: letting the neck be free, letting the head go forwards and up, and allowing the back to lengthen and widen.
3 Continuing to project these directions even while speaking.
4 Just at the moment of speaking, stopping again to reconsider the decision, allowing the freedom not to speak or to do something else.

Psychophysical integrity

As he put what he had learnt into practice throughout his entire daily life, he felt fantastic. He had found a way of managing his body to such an extent that he was in good health, relaxed and moving with a new grace and lightness that he would never have thought possible before. He realized he had beaten his unconscious habits and learnt a new method of being which he called *psychophysical integrity*.

His performances of Shakespeare went from being good to verging on the brilliant. His voice had improved to such an extent that he quickly gained a reputation as one of the foremost Shakespearean actors of his time.

Within a short time he was anxious to pass on his experiences. As people couldn't help but notice the dramatic improvements that he had undergone they were as anxious to learn about this new discovery as he was to teach it. He soon found he had a new, additional career as a voice teacher.

The work

As well as continuing his acting career and teaching voice lessons, Alexander pursued his investigations into the way humans move and operate. He called this *the work* and it was to become his passion and direction for over 50 years.

He quickly developed a considerable following, not only among actors and would-be actors who wanted to develop their talent, but also people sent to him by doctors. The medical profession may have been sceptical at first but Alexander could produce results. Principally he dealt with speech problems but, gradually, he began to see, and treat, a whole range of physical defects.

Slowly he was developing the work into the Alexander Technique. He deliberately chose not to use words and terms that might confuse his clients if they had a preconceived idea of what those terms might mean. He settled for 'the self' and 'in use' rather than 'subconscious' and 'body mechanics'.

The hands-on approach

While all this might seem to have developed quickly, Alexander had actually spent nearly ten years on his work. He started to teach in earnest and found quite often that people didn't understand what he was trying to demonstrate when he merely talked to them about his work. The natural next step was to show his audience his theories by using his hands to move their bodies gently into the right positions. This use of the hands became, and still is today, a fundamental principle of the Alexander Technique but – and this is important – it is not essential. Alexander himself learnt his work through trial and error with nobody using their hands on him. This book will teach you the Technique without you having to spend the same length of time that Alexander did in front of a mirror.

By the turn of the century he was practising in Sydney and had met, and won over, the famous surgeon Steward McKay. McKay suggested that Alexander should go to London if he wanted his work to gain the recognition it deserved. Alexander put on a last farewell tour of *Hamlet* and *The Merchant of Venice*, employing cured patients rather than actors, and then set sail for London in 1904.

Man's supreme inheritance

Once settled in London, Alexander returned to acting at the same time as setting up a practice to teach his work. Within a few years he was known as 'the protector of the London theatre' and could count most of the famous actors of the day, including Sir Henry Irving, among his clients. He subsequently instructed the then Archbishop of Canterbury, as well as Aldous Huxley, Lewis Mumford, George Bernard Shaw, Henry James and many other eminent people. Nineteen doctors signed a letter to *The Lancet* urging that his Technique become recognized and evaluated by their profession because of its remarkable effectiveness in treating many of their patients.

By 1910 there was sufficient interest for unscrupulous people to set up rival practices claiming to teach the Alexander

Technique. Alexander wrote and had published his first book on the subject, *Man's Supreme Inheritance*, in an attempt to set the record straight. This book was to remain in print for the rest of his life.

Off to America

With the outbreak of war in 1914, Alexander took himself off to America where he founded a new practice and for the next decade he spent half the year in America and half in London. His technique was well received and within a short time he had developed a considerably thriving business. Alexander himself was never reluctant to promote his work – his early theatrical training meant that he was still the showman. He was even accused of 'cultism' while in America – an unfounded accusation but understandable because he was the one and only teacher. However, that was to be rectified within a few years.

The first school

The first school was not for people wanting to learn how to teach the Alexander Technique but for small children. In 1924 Alexander set up an infants' school in his studio in London, for children from three to eight, with the intention of teaching them proper *use of self* from an early age. This school ran until it had to be transferred to America in 1940 where it continued to thrive.

The first teacher

The first school for teachers was set up by Alexander in London in 1930, offering a three-year training course. He was absolutely resolute that anyone wanting to teach his work first had to demonstrate that they had learnt, and could exercise, proper use of themselves. Alexander's brother, Albert Alexander, was probably his first trainee teacher. Albert had broken his back in a riding accident and had been told he would never walk again. Alexander taught him about *inhibition*, *primary control* and *conscious direction*. Albert practised in his hospital bed until he was up and moving about. Less than two years after his paralysing accident he was fully recovered and a walking example of the effectiveness of the Technique. He was to remain a lifelong teacher, follower and exponent.

Libel

Alexander's first infant school teacher was Irene Tasker who ran the school for ten years, until she emigrated to South Africa in 1934 where she set up the first independent practice. She had qualified as an Alexander teacher and, with Alexander's approval, was determined to spread the work as wide and as far as possible. This included trying to get it placed on the curriculum of physical education throughout South African schools. The director of the South African Physical Education Committee, Dr Ernst Jokl, was not a devotee, however, and he launched a particularly offensive attack on Alexander, who was left with no choice except to sue for libel.

The case dragged on for many years until, in 1948, Alexander won. The strain of the trial, which he had been unable to attend in person, left him exhausted – he was now nearly 80 – and he suffered a stroke. This was to prove an even greater test than curing his loss of voice. Naturally he used his own Technique on himself and within a few weeks was back teaching and working. He lived for another seven years and died in 1955, aged 86 – not a bad length of life for someone written off as weak and sickly as a child and unable even to attend school.

Spreading the word

During Alexander's lifetime the success of the Alexander Technique was clearly demonstrated. Many eminent doctors and scientists came forward to attest to its remarkable successes. Famous people took lessons and reported widely how effective and reliable it was. On the surface it was a truly extraordinary new development in body awareness and should have attracted a wider following than it did. Part of the reason it didn't was Alexander's own personality. He was not a therapist as we would understand it today – he didn't suffer fools gladly and was quite a tyrant when it came to following the standards he set.

He was also not a conformist and cared little for society. He even moved his mistress into his home with his wife and cared nothing for the scandal it created. He was an inveterate gambler and his love of horseracing sometimes threatened to overshadow his work. He was even declared bankrupt over a debt. He was a forceful person who liked the best that money could buy – good food and fine wines. There was even something of the dandy about him. At times he was dismissed as brash and loud, but he didn't ever attempt to modify or tone down his behaviour. He was a strong individualist and there's no doubt he upset a lot of people. However, viewed with hindsight, he would have fared better in today's climate of media attention and his Technique would have made it on to many a good chat show.

The Alexander Technique today

Since Alexander's death his Technique has gone on quietly growing in strength. Many famous people still attest to its quality, and it is taught in schools and colleges. There are many qualified Alexander Technique teachers, a governing body and a wide following throughout the world. Today you can go to a teacher and have personal lessons, learn about it in books like this one, attend group introductory seminars and listen to Alexander Technique recordings. The Technique's applications are many and varied. It used to be seen as something actors or musicians did to relieve stress and tensions but slowly it has spread as a personal body awareness which teaches you how to manage and use your body well. It is also used as a preventive measure for many body defects such as backache and repetitive strain injury.

Because the Technique is such a personal thing, with sometimes small demonstrable effects, it can become overshadowed by more dramatic therapies and it is probably the most misunderstood of the therapies available – even Alexander himself was hard pushed to come up with a suitable definition, or perhaps he chose not to.

With or without a physical defect to correct, you can learn and benefit from the Alexander Technique purely because it's a method of coping with the unnatural stresses put upon the human frame by the demands of civilized living. This was something Alexander himself was very aware of. Once, when he was explaining his work to his father, his father asked why we should need to learn anything like it when animals managed to perform their physical activities perfectly naturally. Alexander explained that if animals were expected to do half the things we were in a civilized society then they too would need attention. We place unbearable burdens on our bodies by the way we live and, because we grow up with the habit of burden, we don't even realize it – it has come to feel right. We sit in chairs, drive cars, watch television, use stairs, indulge in 'sports', and carry out a million and one unnatural acts that animals don't.

Summary

Alexander developed his Technique as a result of his own problems of voice loss. He saw the cause as threefold:
* he tensed his neck causing his head to go back
* he tightened his throat muscles
* he took a short, deep breath.

He also developed some fundamental principles that can be summed up as:
* the manner of doing – how we develop the habits that precede movements
* not doing – the more we try to correct the faults, the worse we can make it; by not doing we can learn more
* primary control – the relationship between head, neck and torso influences the entire body
* inhibiting – old habits are stronger than the desire to change; before movement we have a choice whether we begin the movement or not.

I expect you'll be anxious to get on and see how all this can affect you. Before you rush ahead – what Alexander called 'end gaining' (we'll learn more about that shortly) – try the following exercises and see if any of the things Alexander discovered apply to you.

Exercises

These exercises are not tests. They are designed to get you thinking about how you hold your body. Don't worry if it all feels uncomfortable and new – we'll sort it all out in the next few chapters.

1 While you are sitting reading this, try folding your arms as you would do normally. How does it feel? Comfortable and relaxed? Now try folding your arms the opposite way – if you normally fold left over right, try right over left. Now how does it feel? Awkward and uncomfortable? Does one shoulder feel higher than the other? When you fold your arms normally one shoulder has to be higher and comfortable. Doing it the other way round is neither better nor worse, right or wrong, it's just different. But because it is not a habit it feels awkward.

2 Now try standing up. Without looking, stand with your feet parallel and about 30 cm (12 in) apart. Now look down and see how accurate you were. Try doing it when you haven't had time to think about it – it's quite common to be either not parallel, or further apart or closer together than you think.

3 Try standing next to a full-length mirror. Without looking in it (keep your eyes closed) adopt a position that feels comfortable. You don't have to stand up straight or anything like that – just relax and stand comfortably. You don't have to be facing the mirror. Now open your eyes and look at yourself. Are you looking as comfortable as you feel? Does your posture appear as relaxed as you thought it was with your eyes closed?

4 Just before you begin to do something – fill the kettle, clean your teeth, etc. – stop before you do it and freeze. Now mentally check your body posture, especially your head and neck. Are you already craning forwards to begin the task? Have you tensed muscles you won't need? Does the position you've frozen in feel comfortable? Could you now decide not to do what you were going to do? Could you now do something else? Could you hold the position you're now in for a while or would it quickly become uncomfortable?

2

what is the Alexander Technique?

We have not learned how to adapt our bodies to modern living – it took a million years for us to adapt to living as humans and we've had only the last 100,000 years to get used to being civilized. Added to this, children are frequently told to 'stand up straight', 'sit up straight', and 'sit still, don't fidget!' However, the response to this usually involves adopting a very unnatural position. For example, standing up straight tends to be done by throwing back the shoulders, sticking the chest out and curving the spine. Sitting still is difficult because human beings are not designed for chairs.

The Alexander Technique is about choices. We sit down and stand up in a certain way because that's the way we do it – we believe we have no choice. Once learned, the Alexander Technique provides conscious choice in everyday activities.

The fundamental things

What I would like to do now is go through with you some of the technical terms and how they apply. This isn't complicated or difficult – it's just that Alexander liked to use new terminology for some of his principles so that there would be no confusion. Some of these terms are, by their very nature, unfamiliar but they are quite easy to understand.

Primary control

Alexander rightly observed that the relationship between the head, neck and torso affects the whole body. If the head and neck are properly aligned with the back, then the whole body naturally follows into a relaxed, natural posture. The problem is that we don't know what properly aligned is – we have never learnt it – and this is probably the vital learning aspect of the Alexander Technique. This problem seems to affect only humans. Are we a design fault? Have we evolved badly? Look at any of the other mammals: cats flow smoothly as they walk; monkeys swing gracefully through the trees; dolphins swim in a perfect streamlined way; leopards run effortlessly. Look at humans and we seem a misconstructed bunch. We sag and walk badly, ache and become unfit. Are we designed to walk on all fours? Or upright on two legs? Left to our own devices we might well spend a lot of the time closer to the ground. We would squat rather than sit in chairs, lounge around on the floor rather than slump on sofas. If you watch children they tend to gravitate towards the floor on most occasions. Parents are forever telling them to 'get up off the floor' as if they're likely to catch some dreadful disease if they lie on the carpet – and yet all they are doing is being, quite naturally, natural.

If you watch soldiers on parade they stand up straight. They are our finest fighting people and should be at their peak of physical fitness. Yet if you watch them they appear stiff and ill at ease.

Alexander said that the head should be directed up and forwards. This direction is not done by deliberately pushing the head into that position but by *consciously projecting*. Once the head is properly aligned, the rest of the body follows.

When we try to stand up straight, or properly, or according to our ideas of 'right', we invariably alter the position of our back, chest or upper torso in some way. Alexander realized that the head leads the entire body posture. Get the head right and the rest will follow suit. Get the head wrong and you'll never be able to do much with the rest of it. However, getting the head right is the most difficult thing to achieve. The reason why most Alexander teachers suggest, quite importantly, that you need lessons on a one-to-one basis is for just that reason – to get the head right.

What's right and what's wrong?

I talk about 'right' and 'wrong' as if there is some overall correct head position. There isn't. There is a right position for you and you alone. We all have different bodies, different heads and different ways of standing, walking, sitting and lying down. To get the head right for all of us using only one position is impossible. All we can attempt to do is get it right for ourselves.

The word *right* is not right. When we talk about right we usually mean good or correct. With the Alexander Technique there is no such thing as 'right' or 'wrong'. There is a *better* position for the head to be in which will allow the rest of the body to become free – but there is no right or wrong. You may know which position is better for you; you may know how to achieve it, and yet you can still choose to stand in a 'wrong' way. Again the whole basis is choice. Something can be wrong only if we do it because we have no choice. Once we have choice we can stand however we like.

How to achieve primary control

Close your eyes and imagine that there is a string attached to the top of your head and it is pulling you gently upright. Just sit for a moment imagining this. As you do so I want you to feel exactly what is happening to your body. I expect you will have imperceptibly moved your head upwards. Your back may have straightened and you will have pulled yourself upright. However, the instruction was to *imagine* what the string was doing.

Now try again knowing, this time, that no body movement is necessary. Just imagine what is happening without moving. Alexander was well aware of the extremely powerful links there are between mind and body. Primary control starts in the mind. If you give your mind an instruction it will subtly control your body.

During the next few days constantly, in different situations, imagine the string pulling you gently upwards. You don't have to do anything. Allow your mind to work on the body at a very subconscious level.

Conscious projection

Alexander, being aware of the close relationship between mind and body, reasoned that if you reprogrammed the mind, the body would automatically follow. However, the reprogramming is the hardest part. Alexander suggested that the way to do it was to repeat constantly specific instructions so that we can hear them as we are moving. The problem with this is that you quickly learn to stop listening – you start to treat the mental directions like a kind of mantra, then you start to feel it is of no value and stop doing it. However, as anyone who has ever used a mantra to meditate will know, the mind operates on a very subtle level. Things are happening when we don't even notice.

Alexander's conscious projections to establish primary control are:

* let the neck be free
* let the head go forwards and up
* allow the back to lengthen and widen.

Again these are not things for you to *do* – they are thoughts for you to think. They are *conscious projections*. You *can* use them like a mantra: repeat them whenever you have a moment to spare; repeat them whenever you sit down, stand up, walk, move, gesture. And every time you find that you are moving as you mentally recite the conscious projection, you should stop and remember that they are only thoughts not actions. We have the thoughts first and the actions follow automatically. There is no need for us to *do* anything. In fact, as Alexander found out – and it took him about ten years – the more we try to do, the worse we will make things.

End gaining

How can trying to do something make it worse? Well, you're being given permission to do nothing. The reason that we let our bodies get into the state that they are in is because we are all doers. Doing causes the problems. When we let go and stop doing we benefit. Not doing is probably the most difficult thing we can do. Humans are great at doing. We build cities, travel to the stars, explore remote continents, climb mountains and drive cars. You name it, we do it. In fact the Hopi Indians of America call Westerners the 'termite people'. We do so much.

This constant doing has created many habits in us. Whenever we have to do something we concentrate on *what* we have to do and not on the *way* in which we do it. End gaining is probably best observed in people in a hurry – maybe they are rushing to catch a train. Their heads will be down and forwards with the rest of the body following on behind at a considerable angle.

End gaining in action

End gaining can be seen in every aspect of our society. The end result is always the most important. We have to get results, and it doesn't matter what we do to ourselves to get those results. It starts as soon as we go to school. Getting exam results is important. We have to look to the future. But I wonder if the quality of our children's education suffers because of end gaining.

We rarely seem to think of how we learn – it's always learning to achieve a result. The scenario seems to be to pass exams so we can go on to higher education to gain a qualification that will enable us to hold down a good job that will see us being promoted higher and higher, because as we rise higher we earn more money and earning more money produces results because we will be happier. Unfortunately for many people, this scenario simply doesn't work. They may end up with the exam, the job, the promotion and even the money – but often it's the happiness they have somehow missed out on.

End gaining is something we all do. Learning how to stop is the key. And we learn by unlearning.

End gaining in our lives

You may like to spend some time working out your own examples of end gaining. How do you rush ahead? We all think to next year's holiday and then when we're on holiday, we think ahead to going back to work.

End gaining is a mental attitude, in which we rush ahead without enjoying the journey. But, as Alexander knew, the mental affects the physical. When we *unlearn* end gaining we can be more relaxed. We'll still arrive, it'll still take the same time to arrive, but maybe we won't be quite so frazzled when we get there. And this applies to every aspect of our lives from the smallest task or journey to the really big things in life, like life and death itself.

The 'means whereby'

End gaining is a habit. Maybe it was once a necessary habit to allow us to survive in caves or when hunting. This habit can be

banish back pain with Alexander Technique

unlearnt, but we need to take apart every movement we make and see why we move in this way. Alexander called this analysis the *means whereby*. How do we *do*? We do by the 'means whereby'. Each action has a means whereby. As we sit, or stand up again, we have a means whereby. Once we start to look at each action needed to complete a task we can begin to question various factors:

* How am I doing this task? – What muscles am I using? How is my body placed? How does it feel? How do the different parts of my body feel in relation to all the other parts?

* Why am I doing this task? – What is the end gain? What will be the result after I have done this task? Why should I continue to do this task? What motivates me to do this task? Is this task suitable for me to do?

Alexander urged his pupils to concentrate on the 'means of the doing', not on the end gain, and by so doing they would naturally relax and move better. When we fail to question the means whereby, we are acting like automatons. When we analyse the means whereby, we start to move like human beings: we are in control and taking responsibility, we are making conscious choices.

Inhibitions

This is Alexander's word for learning to stop just before beginning to do or move. It has come to mean other things since his time, but we will use the word as he meant it – learning to stop.

It's not just about learning to stop, it's about learning to stop to question what we are doing and the means whereby we are going to do it. Inhibition is also an excellent way to avoid end gaining. If every time you are about to rush at something you inhibit first, it gives you a chance to pause to draw breath – to take a little time to become conscious of what you are doing. You can then check the motivation for the task, how it's to be done, what will happen if it's done and how you feel about doing it. These things take only a fraction of a second to do – it's not as if you need to sit down and ponder laboriously for hours. It's just a tiny pause before action while you check that you still want to go ahead and choose the manner in which you want to proceed.

Exercise

You will need a pen and paper for this. I want you to write down exactly how you do three everyday things:

1 How do you get dressed in the mornings? In what order do you put on your clothes? How do you stand or sit while you're doing it? Now I want you to explain, in writing, why you do it like this. You're not allowed to rehearse first – do this entirely from memory.

2 How do you go to sleep at night? How do you get into bed? In what position do you lie? Where exactly is every part of your body? And again, why do you do it like this?

3 How do you make tea/coffee? What do you do while the kettle is boiling? How do you stand? Where is everything positioned? Why?

That's all quite easy, isn't it? Or did you find it hard to remember exactly what you do? It doesn't matter because you're going to do part two of this exercise when it suits you. Put the paper with your details to one side and, when the time comes to do these activities, you can check against what you have written to see how accurate you have been.

After that you can do part three of the exercise which is to repeat the activities, when they occur naturally, and this time inhibit before each and every action. This will give you a pause to check each action to make sure it's what you really want to do. Don't worry at this stage about whether you're doing it right or wrong – just be open to waking up to the fact that you may have been operating unconsciously all your life.

The Alexander Technique is about waking up, questioning what we do, and then finding a better, more efficient, conscious method of doing.

Anti-gravity

The effects of gravity are well known by everyone – everything is continually being pulled down. What may need to be emphasized is how permanent gravity is. It doesn't stop just because we cease to think about it. It's working 24 hours a day, pulling everything towards the centre of the Earth – and that includes us. Every muscle, every tendon, every fibre of our being is fighting gravity all the time. If this wasn't the case, we would be little floppy heaps on the floor. The human body is an anti-gravity entity. It is able to withstand the attacks gravity makes on it for the whole of its life. However, the price that we have to pay is pretty high. Over the years the battle leaves us saggy and stooped. We gradually get beaten down, and although we are never defeated, we can look and feel war-worn and scarred.

Alexander suggests that we could help ourselves become more efficient anti-gravity devices if we were aware of what was going on and had a little help.

Function

Each part of our body has a function. This function is part of its inherent design. The function and its related design are specifically geared to complete certain tasks. Some body parts have a function that is obvious and cannot easily be misused – take your ears for instance. They are ears, they do hearing things and rarely can we use them for anything else. Now take your back. What's its function? What is it actually for? To support the upper part of your body? To lift heavy things? Something clever God thought of to hang the arms on?

Every part has function – and every part has potential function misuse. If we don't know what the correct function is, we cannot correct any misuse.

Stimuli

Suppose someone, a close friend, whom you know really well and respect, comes into the room. They look at you and tell you that they find you stupid, unattractive and rather a waste of space. Imagine how you would react. They've given you the stimulus, now you can have the reaction. You'd probably burst into tears, or run away or shout at them – all of these actions are physical manifestations of stimuli. But remember inhibition. You could take time out to inhibit before you react – and then choose how you will react. You may, having thought about it, choose not to react at all. Your friend smiles broadly and explains it was a joke, a test, they were drunk, whatever.

Suppose every time the phone rings you jump up to answer it. Suppose you're in the middle of something really important – a good argument or making love or having supper – and the phone rings. The stimulus is the ringing sound; what's your response? Most people, not knowing about inhibiting, still jump up and answer it. Now you know about inhibiting you can take a tiny fraction of a second just to question whether what you're doing may be more important – if it is you can choose to continue doing it. Besides which, the answering machine can always react for you, if you have one.

Stimulus is anything that spurs us into action. It could be: emotional – every time we hear a particular piece of music we feel sad; physical – if we hear the phone ringing it makes us jump up; mental – every time I think about all the work I have to do my brain goes cloudy.

Some stimuli set off reactions that are learnt habits and are very difficult not to respond to. I bet we all look when we hear a police siren. We know it's nothing to do with us but we still react whether we want to or not. Sometimes these stimuli are very important, even life saving. In a theatre if someone shouts 'fire' then we need to react. But now we know about inhibiting we maybe don't need to panic – instead we can pause for a tiny moment and choose a more productive response.

Summary

In this chapter we have looked at some of the important terms associated with the Alexander Technique and what they mean. These are:

* primary control
* conscious projection
* end gaining
* the means whereby
* inhibitions
* anti-gravity
* function
* stimuli.

If any of these still feel unfamiliar to you or you're not sure exactly what they mean, it might be worth re-reading this chapter. These terms will be used a lot in later chapters and it will help if you have become familiar with them.

3

what's it for?

As humans evolved it was a necessary part of the process to develop certain defence mechanisms at the same time. The human body, especially the head with its valuable contents, is a very delicate and sensitive piece of equipment that must be protected at all costs. When we lived in caves we had certain responses to danger – responses we still have to this day. These responses are triggered by external stimuli, such as a wild animal approaching, or internal stimuli, such as the pain response that tells us if we need protecting in some other way. However, although these defence mechanisms haven't changed, the world around us has. A lot of common ailments including backache, stress, headache, muscular tension, tiredness, irritability, hypertension, breathing problems, insomnia, stiff neck, 'slipped disc', rheumatism, dietary problems and asthma can be directly attributed to the fact that we use our bodies in a way they were not designed for.

Fight or flight?

When our defence responses are triggered unnecessarily we develop stress patterns that cause muscular tensions throughout the body. The old 'fight or flight' response our ancestors developed is still part of our human make-up, but it is not used nearly as much as it once was. However, we still react to potential danger in the same ways we always have – it's just no longer socially acceptable to fight our enemies physically, or indeed to run away.

Falling down people

So what do we do with all the defence mechanisms the body brings into play when we think we are being threatened? Usually we store them in the form of muscular stress – tensions we learn to live with. And it's the same with the internal stimuli. If every time our body thinks it's going to fall over, it reacts by tensing and preparing itself for injury but then doesn't fall over, it will store that tension as well. The trouble is that, because of the way we have learnt to move, our body thinks it is going to fall over constantly. This chapter is about learning to recognize and eliminate those stored responses. We can't stop the body reacting, but we can change the reaction.

Letting go of excess tension

Before we can let go of any excess tension we have to understand how and why we 'tensed up' and why we continue to hold that tension afterwards. It's all to do with fear. We are frightened most, if not all, of the time. I know you'll be shaking your head at this and disagreeing, so let me explain.

Nature lets us take care of ourselves by incorporating certain reflexes into us. Those reflexes have a very short 'trigger time'. In other words they sit there activated but not actually responding all the time, permanently ready to be switched on whenever there is any hint of danger. It's as if we are living our lives constantly on edge.

In some people the trigger mechanisms are very raw. You probably know people like that: they react by suddenly jumping no matter what – a phone rings and they physically jump. Other people have what appears to be a much more laid-back response time – they don't jump so noticeably. However, they will still react.

There are certain basic symptoms of these reactions. They are usually called the 'startle pattern' and they can be seen physically and be monitored internally.

Symptoms of stress

Physical changes
* head gets pulled down and back
* shoulders raise and hunch
* chest flattens
* arms straighten
* legs bend.

Physiological changes
* blood thickens
* blood pressure increases
* pulse rate increases
* heartbeat speeds up
* digestive system shuts down
* hormones such as adrenalin are released
* arteries constrict.

There are other changes as well that could appear in either list: lungs suck in more air, skin colour changes, temperature drops, sweat glands become activated – even hair will stand on end. All in all, radical changes take place throughout the entire human system. And it happens every time we engage the startle pattern. Can you imagine what it's doing to your body when the phone rings? The startle pattern obviously comes into play to a greater or lesser extent depending on our basic nature, the frequency of and our familiarity with the stimulus, and how we have learnt to cope with stress.

Coping with stress

The Alexander Technique is about learning how we respond, and how we can change some of those responses. You might not be able to control the startle pattern when you are seriously frightened, neither should you want to. All the body changes are very necessary in order to enable us to cope when our lives are threatened. But after the threat, real or imaginary, has departed we hold on to all that tension when we can learn to let go of it. By learning inhibition we can learn how not to respond on such an instinctive level. Taking that micro-second enables us to evaluate the situation. Do we need to react to the maximum? Or could we get away with just a little reflex panic? Should our whole system be put on red alert when the phone rings? Or should we save that for when the wild beasts are coming?

The body needs all the changes if we are actually to fight or run away – all that extra oxygen and blood will be put to good use and the head retracting could save you from a mortal blow. But once the danger is passed we can let go of all the tension. By monitoring our entire system we quickly learn to recognize when we have tensed up and can then deliberately let go.

Falling down again

Obviously a lot of the time the stimuli will be external – road rage, difficult people, unpleasant situations, accidents, disasters and acts of God. But what if we were startling ourselves all the time? Well, I hate to have to be the one to tell you, but we are.

When the external stimuli affect us we can usually see what is going on, but if the stimulus is internal it's harder to detect. What if we think we're falling down and don't even know it? All the body's defence mechanisms would come into play and all we know is that we feel stressed or tired from excess muscular tension.

I called us 'falling down people' because most of us do spend a lot of time falling down but don't realize it. One of the principal lessons in the Alexander Technique is to do with sitting down and standing up. In a lesson, your teacher will spend a lot of time sitting you down and standing you up and you're never quite sure why. Sometimes you seem to get it 'right', but mostly you don't. The reason so much time is devoted to sitting down and standing up is that they are activities that occupy a lot of our waking time, and they are also a good way to really get to understand how and why we tense up.

Internal sensors

Internal sensors detect where and how we are, in terms of balance and space. These sensors haven't evolved at the same pace as our civilizations so they still operate in the same way that our flight or fight responses do, on a primitive level. Basically they tell our brains what we are doing and which muscles we need to be able to do it. When we are standing up we need the big muscles in our back to hold us upright. When we are lying down those big muscles can be turned off as the body knows we are going to sleep. Some of these sensors work by picking up clues from the position of our feet. If our feet are flat on the floor, we are standing up and the muscles get turned on. If our feet aren't touching the floor then we must be lying down and those muscles can be turned off. It's only a two-way switch – on or off – standing up or lying down. That's it and it's simple and it works. So some dumb human had to invent chairs and confuse the whole thing. Sitting is not standing and not quite lying down. As we go to sit down we temporarily lose our balance and for a fraction of a second fall backwards. Result? Yes, all the startle pattern responses come into play and we get very tense every time we sit down to relax. No wonder we're confused.

You might wonder how we used to sit. Well, we didn't. We squatted. This kept our feet flat on the ground so that the big back muscles stayed active and supported us.

Not falling down people

So what can we do about it? We can either stop sitting in chairs and return to squatting, or we can learn to sit down without falling down – and that's easy. Try the following exercise.

Exercise

Try sitting down a few times. Use a hard-backed chair like a kitchen chair. Obviously you have to stand up as many times as you sit down. Each time feel what your head and neck are doing.

Now try it with your hands placed on the back of your neck. Just lightly rest your fingertips there and see what happens now. Does your neck go back? Can you feel yourself tensing? Most people sit by lowering themselves into the chair using their hands or arms and, just as their bottom is about to reach the chair, they let go and fall the last inch or so. This causes the startle reflex and the head goes back and all the other changes we mentioned come into play. You sit and feel worse than before – and that's why.

Try sitting by lowering yourself very slowly – keep your fingertips on the back of your neck – and imagine that someone is about to pull the chair away from under you. You should be able to stop at any moment because at no point do you 'let go'. You keep your balance and don't fall. This means you don't activate the startle reflex so there's no tension and you get to feel relaxed.

It takes some practice because the only way you're going to be able to stand up again is if you let your body fall forwards slightly. Your body will not allow itself to fall and so will propel you forwards and up.

Couch potatoes

It's best if you do the sitting and the standing up exercise from an upright, fairly hard chair. If you try to do it from a sofa you'll have problems. If you want to extend the exercise to include sofas, you'll have to move yourself forwards, from the sitting position, to the front edge of the sofa. That way you'll be in the optimum position to 'fall' upright.

Levering yourself up

This 'falling' upright can be used whenever you have to get up from a sitting position. Two activities that it's worth looking at to see how you do them are getting out of bed and getting out of a car. Again try doing them first as you would normally. Then put your fingertips at the back of your neck and try them again. The fingers on the back of the neck have two purposes: they let you feel all the tension you would normally apply as you get up, and they stop you using your hands or arms to lever yourself up. Levering is what most people do when they want to get up from a sitting position.

What's standing up?

The actual percentage of the human body that needs to be altered to stand is about a third. When you're sitting down you're already two-thirds standing up. Your head, neck and torso are standing up, your lower legs are standing up, it's only your thighs that have to change position – they're the only bits sitting down. By sloping them forwards slightly you're giving them a head start and by using your head to swing yourself forwards and up you only have to pivot your thighs through about 45 degrees. Your head, neck and torso have to move forwards but not change their angle. Your feet and lower legs stay where they are. It's only your thighs that move. It's a simple operation that we all put too much effort into. We don't need to lever ourselves and we don't need to use up valuable energy using the wrong muscles to stand up or sit down.

The two types of muscles

We do in fact have the two types of muscles – voluntary (non-postural) and involuntary (postural). They have different qualities, characteristics, purposes, advantages and disadvantages.

* Voluntary muscles, such as the muscles in your arms and legs, are very flexible; they get exhausted quickly and they need to be directed by you. They are used for manipulation such as fetching, carrying, holding, moving and general duties. Basically they enable us to do things.

* Involuntary muscles, such as the muscles you have in your back, are not very flexible. They can work almost indefinitely and they are 'switched on' by the body's sensors without any input from you. They are used for maintaining the body's posture, resisting tensions and strains, such as when we lift heavy objects, and changing our shape or position. Basically they hold us upright.

The two systems of nerves in muscles

There are two systems of nerves in muscles. We have known about the first system for a long time; it is the system whereby the fibres in the muscles are contracted or shortened. When the nerves stop 'firing', the fibres are relaxed and the muscles lengthen again. The second system has been discovered only recently and it consists of collections of nerves that don't actually go to the muscles themselves but to lots of microscopic bundles buried deep inside the muscles called 'muscle spindles'. They lie alongside the muscle fibres and are responsible for lengthening the muscles. Previously we thought the muscles just relaxed when the first system of nerves stopped firing. Now we know that there is a second process going on as well. The second system could be likened to a fine tuning of the muscles and the spindles have little muscles of their own. They work to prevent the muscles over-contracting when we are using them – a sort of shock absorber.

Dead spindles

When we shorten our muscles continually without relaxing properly, the second system can become inactive and the spindles 'go dead'. This leads to a further shortening of the muscles and the result is poor posture and sagging body form.

The Alexander Technique is about lengthening those muscles again, which in turn reactivates the muscle spindles and allows us to restore full muscle use and activity. People have often said that using the Alexander Technique leads to them feeling fitter and healthier overall, and 'more alive'. It's often the case that because the second system of muscle nerves has been restored to life and is working again, the person feels generally better.

Growing taller

Research by Dr W. Barlow with 50 students at the Royal College of Music in London showed dramatic improvements when they were taught the Alexander Technique. After only six months, 49 of them had increased their height by up to 4.5 cm (1.75 in). The muscle spindles were working again and stopping the muscles, principally the ones in their necks, from over-contracting.

Getting out of the car

The 'levering' that we talked about when standing up is widespread; you only have to watch people getting out of cars. They open the door and grip the edge of the windscreen or the steering wheel to lever themselves upright. A couple of decades of doing that and we have lost most of the strength and use of our involuntary muscles.

Exercise

Use this technique to get out of a car. Open the door of the car, swivel slightly so that your legs are out and then fall upright. Try it and see if it's not easier. You'll be using gravity to work for you rather than against you. The levering is trying to defeat gravity, while the falling is using the weight of your head as a pivot around which the rest of your body weight swivels, until it has reached the upright position.

Confusing your brain

We have seen how the two different types of muscles work. As you go through your day it will be a useful exercise for you to try to see if you use the wrong sort of muscles for various different activities.

Standing up people

Remember, keeping your feet flat on the floor gives your body a good indication of which type of muscle it is supposed to be activating. However, there are several ways of confusing the system. If you sit with both feet flat on the floor, the message being relayed to your brain is that you are a standing up person and it will therefore switch on the postural, or involuntary, muscles and you can sit without getting tired for a long while.

Lying down people

If you then lift your feet up, the message being delivered is that you are a lying down person and the brain will switch off the postural muscles and, if you are going to continue to sit upright, you will need to use the activity, or voluntary, muscles for support. The result of which is that you will get tired quickly. But what happens if you cross your legs? This is where you can confuse your brain dramatically.

Crossing your legs

When you cross your legs, the signals being delivered go haywire and the postural muscles along one side of the body will be switched on, while the muscles on the other side will be switched off. You will then invariably find yourself holding on to something, or propping yourself up in some way. You will sag to one side and need support.

Moral superiority

Again, remember there is no right or wrong way about anything we have discussed. You don't have to sit upright, you can cross your legs when you sit down, you can sag as much as you like. The Alexander Technique is about choice not rules. And it is not about judgement. You may look at someone and think he or she is sitting badly, but it's up to that person and there is no moral superiority in standing 'better'. If it works for you do it, but do it quietly. You may find the Alexander Technique can produce the desired effect if you practise it yourself – telling other people that

they need it or that they are standing badly can put them off
ever wanting to learn about it. If it works for you that's great – let
others wonder about your new graceful way of moving or increased
health and vitality. If they want to know your secret they'll ask, and
you can tell them, but meanwhile just concentrate on yourself.

The three ways of doing

There are only three ways of doing anything:
1 The way you would do it without thinking.
2 The way you would do it if you were thinking.
3 The way it's designed to be done.

Alexander said that the more you try to do it the right way,
the more wrong you'll go. As soon as we have a concept of right or
wrong we are liable to let that concept dictate to us the way we
will stand – and it will be wrong (see Figure 3.1). It might not be the
way we stand that is wrong but the concept most certainly will be.
Because of the way we are brought up we have a concept of what
is right and wrong that is based on false information supplied to
us by others who knew no better themselves. While we hang on to
our ideas of right and wrong we will always get it wrong. When we
let go of our concepts we're in with a chance. We have to look at
'doing' in a fresh way.

The four stages of doing

The Alexander Technique aims to take you from Stage 1 of
doing to Stage 4 of doing. Stage 1 is easy – you're doing it now.
Stage 4 is easy – you were doing it when you were very young.
It's the two stages in between that cause us problems. The four
stages are:
* **Stage 1: unconscious inefficiency** – this is the stage
  you're at – you don't do as you were designed to do
* **Stage 2: conscious inefficiency** – this is the stage you're
  arriving at – you don't do as you were designed to do, but
  you are now aware of it and can see the difference

Misaligned	Misaligned	Aligned
The way you would do it without thinking	The way you would do it if you were thinking	The way it is designed to be done

Figure 3.1 *The three ways of doing (standing).*

* **Stage 3: conscious efficiency** – this is where you begin to do as you were designed to do, but you have to think about it and it feels strange
* **Stage 4: unconscious efficiency** – this is where it all becomes second nature and you again move with the grace and lightness of a child. You move efficiently and don't have to think about it – and it feels 'right'.

So if we're born at Stage 4, how come we end up at Stage 1 and have to relearn everything?

Developing bad habits

As children we learn to walk by falling forwards. Watch any child learning and you will see that each step is a falling into the next step. Children sit on the floor, squat, run around constantly and generally behave quite naturally. Then they go to school and it all starts to go horribly wrong. All their natural instincts to keep moving have to be suppressed and they are told to 'sit still'. They also have to sit in chairs and we've seen how unfortunate that is. Then they have to sit in badly designed chairs and use their voluntary muscles to support themselves. Once learnt, it begins to feel 'right' and they continue that way. If you spend six hours a day as a small child in school being forced to commit your body to unnatural and highly awkward postures it's no wonder you get to believe it must be right. After all, it's the grown-ups who make you do it and surely they must know what they're doing.

All the evidence suggests that children are growing at a faster rate than their parents did – children are taller at a younger age. The chairs and desks, however, haven't changed at all.

Who designed this, then?

If I could change any one of the three problems – sitting, sitting for long periods, and the design of the chairs – it would be the design I would go for. Chairs are not designed to fit humans – they're designed for ease of manufacture.

If you look closely at the way human beings are designed and compare it to the way the chairs are designed there seems to be a fundamental discrepancy. Chairs are hard and angular, invariably the back and seat are at right angles. Humans are soft and rounded with variable angles. Our thighs, when sitting, are not in their most relaxed position if at right angles to our backs. If they are allowed to slope a little they find their most comfortable location. It is also easy to stand up from a position where we are leaning slightly forwards – it makes us keep our feet flat on the floor which helps the internal sensors. If we were to make the front legs of the chair a little shorter than the back legs it would improve things considerably. The position of the head would also be better placed to act as a counterbalance when we stand up. The other problem with chairs is that they come in a uniform size while we don't.

Can you see what the problem is? I don't mean we should all go and chop a couple of centimetres off the front legs of our chairs, I just wanted you to be aware of the problem. You can always use a wedge-shaped cushion to give the same effect. You can make your own by cutting up blocks of foam or you can buy them from a suitable supplier.

It gets worse

Once we've learnt to sit unnaturally and have the unnatural equipment – the chairs – it's only a matter of time before we sag. The teacher comes around and tells us to 'sit up straight'. This we do by arching our back and throwing our chest forwards. It seems to do the trick because the teacher moves on to sort someone else out.

Maximum points for bad backs

As children we are told that an unnatural body posture earns us maximum points. So what do you think happens next? That's right, we adopt that unnatural posture whenever we want to impress, avoid trouble, receive praise, earn points, whatever. How many times were you told to stand up straight?

During our teen years slouching is a sign of indolence or rebellion, while standing up straight is to do with conformity and thus goodness. By the time we reach our twenties the conditioning has gone in hard and deep. Not only do we not know how to place our bodies, but we don't even know that we don't know.

Summary

Why should we ever have thought anything was wrong? Alexander was lucky in the sense that he had voice loss to point him in the direction of something being not right with his body. But us? It ain't broke – why should we do anything?

It may not be broke, but I bet it's getting pretty close to it by now. Ever had backache, stress, headache, muscular tension, tiredness, irritability, hypertension, breathing problems, insomnia, stiff neck, 'slipped disc', rheumatism, dietary problems, asthma?

A lot of common ailments can be directly attributed to using our bodies in a way that they were not designed to be used. The next chapter is about who can benefit from the Alexander Technique, but to summarize this chapter we learnt about:

* responses to stress
* letting go of excess tension
* the startle pattern
* the body's defence mechanisms
* internal sensors
* the two types of muscles
* the two systems of muscle nerves
* confusing the system
* the four stages of doing
* developing bad habits.

4

who can benefit from it?

Originally Frederick Alexander developed his technique for himself as a curative process to eliminate his constantly recurring problem of voice loss as an actor. Once he had diagnosed the cause of the problem, he went on to investigate all aspects of muscular control and tension elimination. However, his primary and overriding objective was to *cure* something that was wrong. Today the Alexander Technique is promoted mainly as a system of learning good body use and as a means of promoting health. But it is important to remember that it was originally developed as a curative discipline – and it still works well as such today. Everyone can benefit from the Alexander Technique, and once the Technique has been learned it can be applied to new situations as they occur, changed and adapted, and constantly monitored as it is put it into practice. It's an operating system which can help you to operate efficiently.

Suitable candidates

So who can learn the Alexander Technique? Basically, anyone. You don't even have to be convinced that it will do anything for you – I certainly wasn't to begin with. In fact, I didn't know anything about it, not even what it was called. I just knew it worked. You may come to it because you have heard about it and are just interested, or you may have a major problem that has so far resisted all attempts by orthodox methods to be remedied and want to try something new, or you may even be sceptical. Whatever, your motivation, it is worth learning – it works.

Combining lessons

I assume you are interested or you wouldn't have got this far with this book. Learning it yourself works well but if you have a particular problem, like backache, then it's probably best if you combine self-teaching with a course of individual lessons. There's nothing quite like having an Alexander teacher give you all that time and attention as well as helping you to correct things that have been wrong for a long time and you have not been able to resolve before. It's a nice feeling. Sometimes it's useful to have a refresher lesson just to check that you've still got the simplicity behind the Technique correct. It's so easy to add on and complicate things without even really trying. It may also be useful to have the odd lesson after reading a book such as this one. After all, what I write and what you read may turn out to be two different things. It's always useful just to check that we've both got it right. You could even attend one of the regular workshops on the Alexander Technique that take place.

Suitable cases for treatment

The Society of Teachers of the Alexander Technique (STAT) says that the Alexander Technique 'addresses the fundamental causes of many cases of back pain, neck and shoulder tension, breathing disorders, stress-related illnesses and general fatigue where misuse and a loss of poise are contributory factors'. Many teachers have found that it is beneficial in treating a wide range of ailments – often these 'clear up' as a side effect or bonus.

The Alexander Technique is beneficial for many ailments – both physiological and psychological – including:

* muscle fatigue
* migraine
* depression
* high blood pressure
* stress-related disorders including ulcers, eating disorders and digestion problems
* circulatory problems
* backache problems
* respiratory problems, e.g. asthma
* speech defects.

There are many other problems, complaints and disorders that people have that can benefit from the Alexander Technique. There's no need to list detailed case histories here – we are all different and what affects someone with a particular complaint may not affect others in the same way. How are we supposed to be? Fit, active and healthy. If we're not, then let's try to change it.

Freeing ourselves from illness

Practising the Alexander Technique allows us to harmonize our bodies, minds and emotions. Once we have this harmony, we are more able to free ourselves from illness. There is an old Chinese saying: 'In the West when something happens they ask what they can do about it – here in the East we ask what caused it.' The Alexander Technique is a way of looking at what causes our bodies to malfunction. Invariably, it's because we didn't know how they were supposed to function in the first place. Once we learn how we are supposed to be, we can practise it.

Let's see how body shape can affect respiratory problems.

1 Scrunch yourself up as tight and as tense as you can, pull your head down into your body and shorten and tense your neck, clench your fists with your arms pressed tightly across your chest. Now take the deepest breath you can and see how long you can hold it. Let it out and say 'ahhh' as you do so.

2 Now let go of all that tension, allow your body to lengthen and widen, head up and out, arms loosely by your side, smile. Now take the deepest breath you can and hold it. Let it out and say 'ahhh' as you do so.

3 Compare the two results. In 1 the deep breath is nowhere as deep as in 2, and the time you can hold that deep breath is much shorter. Also, in 2 the 'ahhh' is deeper, richer, more resonant that in 1. How can you breathe properly if you're tense and scrunched up?

Your approach

Some Alexander Technique teachers report quite staggering results with arthritis, rheumatism and asthma, often as an unlooked for bonus. If you suffer from any of these conditions and they have not responded to orthodox treatments, or you wish to check out a more natural method, then seeing a qualified Alexander teacher can do you no harm. Learning the Technique can only improve your basic body poise and that is something we can all benefit from. Expecting dramatic results is probably not the best way to approach the Alexander Technique – it's too subtle for that. It's best to adopt a 'try it and see' approach. Then, when it works, you'll be delighted. But if the effects are relatively small, you will be more philosophical than disappointed.

Healthy teeth

The benefits of the Technique can have far-reaching effects that we wouldn't even think of. If I told you that the health of my teeth has improved, you'd probably think I was imagining it. However, it's a fact that was pointed out to me by my dentist – and she didn't even know I was doing (or not doing) anything. Quite simply, I had learnt to question the way I did *everything* and I was experimenting with trying to change my habits. I noticed that I was always brushing my teeth by leaning on the basin with my left arm, bending over, tensing up, and twisting slightly to the right while I brushed vigorously with the toothbrush in my right hand. The only way I could stop myself hanging on with my left arm, a totally unproductive exercise, was to swap hands. I tried brushing my teeth holding the brush first in one hand and then the other. It felt very strange so I knew I was on to something. Anyway, you know the rest. Using a different hand to hold the toothbrush meant I was cleaning the back teeth on the lower right side of my mouth better than they had ever been cleaned before: less decay and thus fewer fillings. An unexpected bonus indeed.

Improving performance

Alexander, being an actor, naturally promoted his new discoveries amongst fellow entertainers. Musicians latched on pretty quickly, followed by athletes and dancers. Today, anyone who uses their body in complicated habitual manoeuvres can benefit, and that includes just about all of us. Learning how to do what we do with a new poised posture can only be helpful.

Wasting energy

If every time we move we expend valuable energy it makes sense to move with minimum effort – wasting energy is not only exhausting, but also unproductive. If this sounds a little serious you may like to look at it another way: all the energy you later save can be used for activities you really like. Why waste energy sitting down and standing up when you could save it and spend it later doing something much more interesting?

The three types of candidates

Basically, I see people who want to learn the Technique as being one of three types:

* people who want to learn it in the hope it will alleviate a specific condition or complaint
* people who want to learn it to help improve a particular thing they do with their bodies, like dancers or musicians
* people who want to learn it for general interest.

Occasionally you do get someone who doesn't fit into any of these categories. At one introductory workshop I was running I asked all the people there why they were attending. Everyone fitted into one of the three categories except one woman who was strangely reluctant to reveal why she was there. With a little gentle probing I got to the real reason, and it's nothing horrendous. It was merely that she was a journalist from a national newspaper, who'd been sent along to find out what it was all about. She wrote her article and still practises regularly.

At another workshop, again everyone fitted into the three categories except one woman. Why was she there? Quite simple, she explained, the Alexander Technique was the only therapy she hadn't yet done. A therapy collector.

End gainers and A types

We talked earlier about end gaining and you may already know about A and B types. In case you don't, here's a brief summary:

* **A types** – impatient, aggressive, ambitious, hurrying, rushed, quick, stressed, demanding, difficult, loud, creative, leading, rousing, dynamic, confident, decisive.
* **B types** – patient, defensive, relaxed, considerate, cautious, careful, following, receptive, caring, nervous, questioning, indecisive, quiet, philosophical, thorough.

Which are you?

I'm sure you can add many more attributes to both lists. Which type are you? Probably a good mixture of both, but most of us want to be more B than A. We all know that B types live longer, suffer fewer heart problems, less stress, fewer frustrations and setbacks, because they think things through more, have a calmer outlook, are more laid-back and are generally nicer people. But A types can have more fun living on the edge, more excitement, are better at solving (and probably causing) problems, exploring, discovering, creating and leading. I have no desire to give up my A-ness, I just want to be less end gaining about it. The Alexander Technique allows us to be ourselves without having to change our basic personality (though we can if we want to – it's all to do with choice). Sometimes we need A types around and sometimes B types. I wouldn't like to be facing danger with a B – that's the time you need an A.

B types have their downside, too. They appear to be more prone to the ill effects of carcinogens, more prone to neurosis and mental disorders, less likely to achieve or 'reach the top', more prone to worry and sleep disorders, and more prone to dietary disorders and respiratory problems.

Living with the two types

We are what we are, there's no better or worse. I have two sons, one an A and the other a B. I tend to think of them as Mr Bouncy and Mr Book. There is no way I love either more or less. Each is different and equally wonderful. They will both go through life encountering their own set of problems and solving them in the way they are uniquely equipped to do. Mr Bouncy will rush at everything and keep doing so until the problem is resolved. Mr Book will think long and hard, and eventually the problem will go away of its own accord. Each way creates its own problems and each way works – for them. (I also have a daughter, but she's an O type – 'Oh, Dad, I need more money; Oh, Dad, I haven't got enough clothes; Oh, Dad, I need a lift!')

Changes to your basic personality

If you think I've gone on a lot about this, it's because the Alexander Technique requires you to make no changes to your basic personality. It's fine to be who you are: you'll just be moving more gracefully while being you. You don't have to give up anything except your tension. You don't have to believe any philosophy, you just have to try it. If it works, do it; if it doesn't, don't. You don't have to believe anything, it's all subject to testing and results. A types will ask, 'What can this do for me?'; B types will want to know, 'How will it make me feel?'

How A types will benefit

A types will benefit because they, by becoming more relaxed and expending less energy, can get more done. They will be able to move faster, be less clumsy and suffer fewer accidents. They will be able to pace themselves better and not have to recover quite so often.

How B types will benefit

B types will benefit because they will feel fitter and healthier and more in harmony. They will increase their understanding of themselves, have a valuable insight to share with their friends and families and be more dynamic because of their increased energy levels. They will be more confident, poised and capable.

Taking responsibility

There is a tendency in the West to blame our problems on others: we can't get on because we're being held back; if only so and so was nicer to us we'd be happier; if only you loved me more my life would be better; it's all your fault I'm the way I am. Once you take responsibility for your body you take responsibility for your outlook. Alexander knew full well the vital connection between body poise and emotional well-being. It's no good blaming everyone for the shape we're in. No amount of blaming will alter it one tiny bit. Even if you could gather all your teachers together and tell them off and they were to all confess their faults and apologize to you, you would get not one jot better. You are who you are now, and only you can effect change. By not blaming, and instead taking responsibility for who and how we are, we can make positive changes. Once we make those changes our outlook improves: we are already improving because we are making changes. It's a non-vicious circle, a benign upward spiral if you like.

Treating depression

The more we blame, the less we do about it. I have seen some very dramatic improvements in people suffering severe depression when they've been taught the Alexander Technique.

Simple test

So you may be asking if you can benefit. Simple test – stop reading and go and find a full-length mirror. Take all your clothes off and have a look at yourself sideways. If there's anything in your posture that you're not happy about, you can change it. Yes, you can benefit.

Exercise

First adopt the classic 'depressed' body shape – allow your shoulders to hunch, drop your head, frown and pull your mouth down at the corners, tense your whole body inwardly as if expecting a blow, and say out loud 'I feel absolutely miserable'. Now you know why it's called depression – you have just physically depressed your entire body.

Now let all that tension go and adopt the 'happy' posture – head up, smile, open body shape, relaxed, confident, and say out loud 'I feel fantastic!'.

Now try adopting the depressed posture and say out loud 'I feel fantastic!'. Then adopt the happy posture and say 'I feel absolutely miserable'. See what happens. When we physically depress ourselves we feel depressed. When we physically open up, so do our feelings. It's almost impossible to feel happy if our bodies are shut down and it's a whole lot easier to feel less depressed if we're not physically depressed.

What makes the Alexander Technique so different?

The Alexander Technique is not therapy or a discipline. I like to think of it as an operating system. An analogy I use is that it's a bit like having a computer. You have to have *software* (your programs, such as a word processing package or some games to play) and you have to have some *hardware* (your screen, keyboard, printer and CPU – the big box that contains the central processing unit that sits on your desk), and you have to have an *operating system* (usually called something like MS-DOS – the system that tells your computer how to set itself up, which language to speak, what to do when you turn it on and how to load and use the software). Well, therapies or disciplines or whatever we do are the software, your body is the hardware and the Alexander Technique is the operating system. The one we normally have is built out of bits at random, bits left over from childhood, school, wherever. By learning a new operating system we link the hardware and software together to work efficiently. In normal use you don't see the operating system, and so it is with the Alexander Technique. Once installed it should not be visible.

How the Technique fits in with other disciplines

You can use the principles of the Alexander Technique to improve any other activity you do. A question often asked is, 'Which should I learn, the Alexander Technique or something like tai chi or yoga or aerobics?' Well, you can use the principles of the Alexander Technique when you're learning, say, tai chi and you'll find them helpful and they definitely add something. I'm not sure it works the other way round. I would suggest that the Alexander Technique is something you learn first, then you can learn any of the others and do them well. If you learn the others first you may well be doing them in a way that isn't completely efficient right from the start. If you already practise another discipline, try to apply some of the principles you're learning here and see if it changes anything.

The Alexander Technique also works well with other complementary therapies. For instance osteopaths, chiropractors and massage therapists will often refer clients for the Alexander Technique.

Summary

It's taken a lot to answer the question posed by this chapter. I think the short answer to the question 'Who can benefit from it?' is: you, me, anyone, everyone, all of us.

And it's not just something we learn, get good at and then think we've done it. Alexander took ten years developing it, taught it for over 50 years, and it was said that he did his best work in the last five years of his life. He was still developing it to the very end.

Once you've learnt the Technique you can apply it to new situations as they occur, change and adapt it as you change and adapt in your life, constantly monitor it as you put it into practice, use it to refresh yourself whenever you feel you're going back into old habits, and find new ways to incorporate it into your daily life. It's an operating system: once learnt it just sits in the background helping you to operate efficiently.

5

how is it done with guidance?

Frederick Alexander learned and knew his Technique better than anyone else has ever done, yet he never had a single lesson in his life. So how important are lessons? The Society of Teachers of the Alexander Technique (STAT) advocate lessons as being very important. It is useful to have lessons to correct a particular fault or to check you are using the Technique properly. Some people keep their lessons going on a regular basis for years. Others have one or two and then find they have learned enough to help them. It's up to individuals and their teachers to decide what is appropriate. Lessons should only be taken from qualified STAT-approved teachers. To qualify as a member of STAT, teachers have to complete a three-year training course approved by the Society or one of the affiliated societies overseas to reach a standard that the Society considers competent.

Watching yourself

I believe that you can, like Alexander himself, learn a great deal from watching yourself. Probably the best approach is to learn all you can from books so that you have a thorough grounding in the principles and then have some lessons to make sure you're putting it all into practice as efficiently as possible. The number of lessons you take can be discussed with your teacher and depends on your particular needs and goals. I've found that lessons help me correct specific faults and learning from books has given me an understanding of how it works, but the most I've learnt has certainly been from self-observation. Lessons work well during the actual lesson, but if you're anything like me you'll forget everything you were shown the minute you walk out of the treatment room. I can do anything with perfectly relaxed poise when I want to demonstrate or impress: it's much more difficult when I have to apply it all unconsciously or when I encounter new situations like waking up in hospital.

What does it cost?

STAT advises that lessons should cost (at the time of writing this book) £25–40.

Some insurance providers such as WPA, Universal Providence and Medicash cover the cost of lessons when they have been recommended by a consultant as part of a treatment plan. In some cases the NHS funds lessons.

A typical lesson

Let's run through exactly what happens when you go for your individual lesson. Let's suppose you have chosen a qualified teacher, made your first appointment and arrived at their place of teaching. You don't have to wear anything special, although loose, light clothing like a tracksuit is suggested, as anything tight and heavy restricts not only your movements, but also your teacher's observations of you and how you move. You will not need to remove any clothing for the lesson.

Disturbing questions?

The teacher will not ask you any probing or disturbing questions about your childhood, sex life or lifestyle, so you don't have to worry about revealing anything you may be embarrassed about, or reluctant to discuss. You may be asked in a general way what you do and if you're a family person. That's partly so that the teacher can get an idea of what sort of person you are and what sort of routine you might have. It's more likely to be general conversation designed to relax you and put you at ease. The teacher doesn't need to know anything about you, except how you move. Anything else you choose to tell your teacher is entirely up to you, it can be as much or as little as you want.

Medical history and medication

I would suggest that if you have any physical disability or complaint you should tell your teacher in advance. You may have a particular medical history that precludes you from having lessons. If you're not sure, discuss it with your teacher and/or your doctor. And if you are receiving any medication you should check with both your teacher and your doctor that having lessons will in no way interfere with your treatment.

Ask any questions you want to – they should be answered easily and openly. The Alexander Technique is suitable for people of all levels of physical fitness.

Your first lesson

The first few minutes of your first lesson will probably be spent chatting. This helps put you at your ease and lets you and your teacher get to know each other. Most teachers will then ask you to stand up or sit down while they place their hands gently on your neck. This is so they can feel how tense you are, how you perform simple movements and so that you get used to them touching you.

Some people find it quite emotionally uncomfortable to have a stranger touch them, even in this sort of a way.

Your teacher may well give you a short introductory talk about what the Alexander Technique is – or rather isn't. So many people go to their first lesson full of concepts of how it's about posture and standing up straight. Teachers often say that it takes longer to re-educate people than to educate them in the principles of the Alexander Technique.

Your teacher may ask you to carry out some simple movements such as sitting down and standing up, lying down and getting up, walking up and down. They will probably ask you to do these several times. The first few times you will be conscious of them watching you, you may even try to do them 'properly', but eventually you relax, forget that the teacher is there and just do them in the same old way you would at home. Then your teacher can see how you really move. You may be asked to stand with your back against a wall. This is so that the teacher can see how your back is shaped. All in all, you'll be thoroughly observed and won't notice at all.

Your teacher may ask about any accidents or injuries you've had during your life. You've probably forgotten most of them, so it may be helpful if you spend some time before the lesson making a note of them.

The semi-supine position

Your teacher may ask you to lie in the semi-supine position. Basically you lie on the floor on your back with your knees bent and some hard books under your head. This position, when adopted properly, encourages your back to lengthen and widen as well as correcting your head–neck relationship. The semi-supine position allows maximum support and relief for the back.

While you are lying in the semi-supine position, your teacher may place your arms, head and legs in a slightly different position from the one you are in. They are straightening you out. It may feel odd or awkward but you can trust them. Standing above you they can see much more clearly how straight you're lying. They are also trained to do this.

If your teacher does move you, go with the movement. Don't resist. If you are resisting, your teacher may ask you to 'give me the weight'. This means that you should go completely limp. Be like a dead thing: no resistance, no tension, no thought of where you're supposed to be placing your body. Let your teacher do it; they're trained, qualified and being paid to do it. You just relax and enjoy the experience of realizing that you haven't got a clue what you 'should' be doing, what you 'think' you should be doing, or even whether you should be doing anything at all.

Little monkeys

You may well be shown the classic *monkey* stance, or *position of mechanical advantage* to give it its technical name. Essentially, you'll be shown how to stand bending slightly from the hips and with your knees also slightly bent. This teaches you about the most efficient head–neck–back relationship.

Hands on

Your teacher may well stand you up and sit you down several times while keeping one hand on the back of your neck and the other on the top of your head. As you stand up and sit down your teacher will make minute adjustments to the position of your head and neck. During a course of lessons the 'feel' of where your head is supposed to be becomes more natural, although at first it will feel quite strange.

Ahhh

If your teacher asks you to breathe out while making an 'ahhh' sound, this isn't to check your tonsils or vocal chords. It's to get you to let your ribcage expand. This allows the back to lengthen and widen. The 'ahhh' sound also teaches you what a loose jaw feels like and a loose jaw is a relaxed jaw. Many people hold their jaw extremely rigid. Making the 'ahhh' sound as you breathe out relaxes most of your face as well. As you make the sound you are encouraged to smile – more relaxation. The 'ahhh' is not spoken with the vocal chords, but rather the sound of the breath coming out of your mouth as you release all the tension you are holding.

Other practices

You may be asked to kneel, crawl, squat and even run. It all depends on the individual teacher and how they think you need directing and correcting. You may even be asked to adopt the Muslim prayer position. No, not to pray, but so you can feel what's happening to your back.

Different strokes for different folks

Individual teachers may have other exercises and positions I haven't mentioned here. Your lesson will be tailored to suit you and, as such, may be very different from what anyone else has or doesn't have. There's no point comparing with anyone else. There's not a lot of point competing either. The only way of monitoring your progress is by how you feel.

Homework

You may be given exercises to practise at home in between lessons. You will be given directions – conscious projections – to say to yourself as you go about your daily tasks. These will probably be: let the neck be free; let the head go forwards and up; allow the back to lengthen and widen.

Subsequent lessons

Your follow-up lessons will usually be much the same as the first lesson. You may think you've got the Technique just right only to keep being corrected every time you go for a lesson. Then, when you're convinced you've got it wrong, your teacher will tell you that you've got it right.

The teachers

Alexander teachers are ordinary people, like you and me, who have decided to make being a teacher of the Alexander Technique their profession. You should treat your appointment in the same way you would treat a visit to your doctor, dentist, osteopath or whoever. Keep your appointments, arrive on time, pay their fees on time and treat them in a professional manner. This also means that they are working for you. If you are unhappy or have a complaint then tell them, and expect them to accommodate your needs. If you continue to be unhappy with the service provided then change your teacher. You don't have to stick with a teacher you don't particularly get on with, either. They, like us, are all different. You may find one you really relate to straight away. You may find you need to try several before making your final choice. Listen to other people's recommendations. Go to introductory courses. Get the list of qualified teachers from STAT. Shop around until you're satisfied, and then go for it. The Alexander Technique teaches natural body poise: it's not a therapy or a religion or a cult or a 'new age' manipulation process. It's a professional learning method, a science, if you like, taught by teachers who belong to an extremely professional governing body. These professional teachers have to be approved by the Society.

How do you get approved as a teacher?

To qualify as a member of STAT, teachers have to complete a three-year training course approved by the Society or one of the affiliated societies overseas to reach a standard that the Society considers competent. The course is full time and the teachers have to abide by the Society's published code of professional conduct and competence. It costs teachers around £12,000 to complete the course so they have to be dedicated.

Who's suitable?

Applications for teacher training are invited from individuals who are already committed to learning the Alexander Technique for their own personal development. Since Alexander teachers are often called upon to work with people of widely differing ages, needs and interests, almost any form of previous training and experience can be an advantage, but none is essential. Prior experience of lessons would usually be expected. I suggest you telephone the school you wish to attend.

Course content

During their three-year course, students work in small groups with their course instructor. Their work is mainly of a practical nature but time is given for lectures and discussions on basic anatomy, physiology, the Technique itself, practical demonstrations and other related topics.

In their final year, students work under supervision on fellow students and sometimes on members of the public. They are monitored throughout their course in their own use and understanding of the Alexander Technique. By the time they get to you they know their subject well.

Workshops and introductory groups

As more and more people get to hear about the Alexander Technique there has been an increased demand for STAT to organize some way of explaining what it is about to interested people. They arrange for qualified teachers to demonstrate and explain the Technique at introductory workshops and it may be useful for you to attend one. You don't have to pay for a course of lessons, but you do get to see the Technique being demonstrated in a practical way.

These workshops are usually one-day introductory courses and they take place in all sorts of places throughout the world. You can contact them in your country and they will give you all the information you require regarding where and when workshops are scheduled. For the United Kingdom you need to contact their London headquarters. You can also learn the Alexander Technique under the auspices of the local education authority in some areas. You need to check with your town hall or library to see if workshops or classes are available in your area.

How widespread is the Alexander Technique?

To give you some idea, there are approximately 840 teaching members of STAT in the United Kingdom alone. There are teachers in many European countries as well as Brazil, Israel, Africa, the United States, Canada, Australia and New Zealand. Worldwide there are approximately 3,000 members, and STAT is the internationally recognized governing body.

There is also a registered charity Friends of the Alexander Technique open to all interested individuals. It is an organization for people who use the Alexander Technique in any aspect of their lives.

Summary

Have lessons if you need to correct a particular fault or to check you are using the Technique properly. Some people keep their lessons going on a regular basis for years. Others have one or two and then find they have learnt enough to help them. It's up to you and your teacher to decide what you need. Have lessons only from a qualified STAT approved teacher if you feel you want lessons, but remember Alexander himself never had a single lesson in his life. Anyway, that's enough about lessons – it's time you learnt more about how to do it for yourself.

6

how to do it for yourself

There are three stages to the Alexander Technique: inhibitions, conscious projection and primary control. The term 'inhibitions' refers to stopping and thinking before making a movement; 'conscious projection' is an instruction to yourself regarding a movement; and 'primary control' refers to the positioning of the head. It is important to fully understand these three stages before the Technique can be put into practice. One of the first steps in practising the Technique is to look at how the body is being used, and what effect that is having. Even our emotions can influence the way we move. Often, we will find that we are out of alignment and aren't using our bodies in the way they have been designed for. Once unhelpful habits have been identified, we can find new ways of doing everyday tasks, such as walking and sitting, that can enable us to make the best use of ourselves.

Many people have put forward definitions of the Alexander Technique. However, it is said you have to experience it to understand it. The following are all definitions of the Alexander Technique from teachers, authors and psychologists.

* A system of postural re-education and good body use.
* General improvement in the use of the body from which correction of individual detailed faults will follow.
* A means for changing stereotyped response patterns by the inhibition of certain postural sets.
* A method for expanding consciousness to take in inhibition as well as excitation and thus obtaining a better integration of the reflex and voluntary elements in a response pattern.
* A method of posture training.
* A technique by which mind and body are harmonized.
* Learning to move your joints and muscles correctly.
* A series of physical movements designed to correct bad posture and bring the body back into alignment, thus helping it to function efficiently, as nature intended.

It's interesting to look at what Alexander himself had to say when asked to sum it up. He said: 'How can you name something which is so comprehensive. If you do what I did, you'll be able to do what I do.' And what he did was to consciously examine every movement he made and then analyse why and how. Once he was aware of the movement, he learnt to *inhibit* to prevent the old habits controlling the movements and then to substitute new controls – *conscious projections* – to replace the habits, and then to move using *primary control* – allowing his head and neck to be free and properly aligned. Those essentially are the three stages of the Alexander Technique. Now we have to learn how to put it all into practice.

Misconceptions

Before we begin, I would like to clear up a few popular misconceptions that arise around any teaching of the Technique:

* **Inhibitions** – These are nothing to do with the Freudian concept of suppressed or repressed emotions. Inhibitions, in Alexander terminology, means stopping and thinking before making a movement to give yourself a chance to change your mind and not continue with the movement, or to continue, or to do something else. The inhibition is done before any movement has taken place. It's a tiny pause before you move while you consider the value of the movement.

* **Conscious projection** – This is not a meaningless mantra to be repeated to dull or empty the mind. It is a conscious instruction to yourself before you make a movement and while you are making it. The conscious projection is: let the neck be free, let the head go forwards and up, allow the back to lengthen and widen. Conscious projection is a thought; it is not a movement of any sort whatsoever. You think it, you don't do it. You are letting and allowing. This is not movement, it is permission.

* **Primary control** – The head should be directed up and forwards. First: up is not a place, it is a direction. It is the direction that the top of the spine happens to be pointing in. When you're sitting or standing, up is towards the ceiling; if you are lying down up is towards the head of the bed; if you were crawling, up would be towards the wall in front of you. Second: directing the head forwards does not mean you thrust it forwards. Forwards, again, is a direction. You tilt your head, where it balances on top of the spine (between the ears, not the top of the neck), until it is directed forwards.

Please read and re-read these three points until they are fully and instinctively understood. They are probably the most important aspect of learning the Technique. We can go no further until they are second nature. However, as Alexander said, 'We can throw away the habits of a lifetime in a few minutes if we use our brains.'

Are you aligned?

After all these years of not making proper *use* of yourself, you may be *out of alignment*. If you were having lessons it would be one of the first things your teacher would look for. So how do you know whether you're out of alignment? Try this simple exercise. Find yourself an area of blank wall. You should be wearing light clothes, or no clothing at all, and be barefoot. Stand with your back to the wall and position your feet so that they are 46 cm (18 in) apart with your heels 5 cm (2 in) out from the wall. I suggest that you actually measure these two measurements and mark them on the floor. It's easy to get them wrong when you're looking down at your feet from above.

At first, don't touch the wall at all. Then relax and let yourself lean gently back against the wall. If you are well aligned your shoulder blades and buttocks will touch the wall all at the same time. These are your *three points of reference* (see Figure 6.1).

If one shoulder blade touches before another, then you are slightly twisted or *one-sided*. If your buttocks touch first, you are holding your pelvis too far back. If your shoulders touch first, you are holding your pelvis too far forwards.

Now you're leaning back, can you feel what is touching? I bet there's a big gap between your lower back and the wall.

Try this exercise every morning when you first get out of bed and again last thing at night. It will encourage the realignment of the body.

Help! I'm out of alignment

First of all, don't panic. We're all out of alignment to some extent and we can put it right. If you find that there's that gap between your lower back and the wall, try bending your legs at the knees slightly until the gap disappears – you will have to slide down the wall a bit (see Figure 6.1). Let your arms hang loosely at your sides and don't *do* anything. Stay like this for a

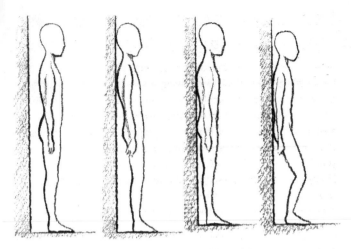

Figure 6.1 *Leaning against a wall – four stages.*

while. This is a useful exercise for correcting misalignments, but only if you actually do it. Gradually, over a period, you will find that you touch the wall at all three reference points at the same time and the gap will go. If you still touch one shoulder blade first, you are allowed to *untwist* so that you are touching at all three points.

You may find that the feeling of standing with your back to the wall, without your knees bent, can be quite strange – it feels as if you are leaning backwards. However, I can guarantee you that you are standing more upright than you have for a long time. It's all to do with the centre of gravity. It's never where we think it is. More about that later.

If you are out of alignment you may find standing with your knees bent fairly uncomfortable to begin with. Persevere – it will get easier, I promise you. I suggest you try this a few times to get to know how you feel and then incorporate it into a routine of exercise to correct matters. You can use the time to remember the three vital points – inhibit, project, control. Do them as you stand there, do them as you lean backwards, do them as you correct your alignment.

How did I get out of alignment?

I don't know how *you* personally got out of alignment – we are all different and all end up in a similar situation although we may arrive by different routes. There may, however, be a few things we all have in common.

Stand against the wall again, with your legs straight and now lift your heels a couple of centimeters (an inch) off the ground. What happens to your alignment? Try doing the exercise as before right from the start, but this time do it on tip-toe. What happens now? You'll probably find it quite hard to touch your buttocks against the wall without bending your knees or contorting your back. That's the effect you get every day when you wear shoes with heels on them. Now, can you explain why we wear shoes with heels? We don't need them, so what's it all about? I don't know the answer to any of these questions but you might like to think about them while you're standing against the wall. Why are all kitchen units a standard height when we're not? Why are most beds a standard height? Why are chairs, stairs and steps all a standard height? Why are train seats so uncomfortable? Why are the foot pedals in cars where they are?

The two parts of the Technique

Any teaching of the Technique has to be divided into two parts; both have to be learnt and practised simultaneously. In a book we can progress only in a linear fashion so we have to work through the points separately.

What we are doing and the way we are doing it

First, we have to find out *what* we are doing and whether the *way* we are doing it is efficient and fits in with the body's design. And then we look at *how* what we are doing affects us. In other words, find the habits, find how we do them and check what they are doing to us.

The best use of ourselves

Second, we have to find new ways of doing that make the best *use* of ourselves, doing efficiently and according to the best features of the body design. And stop the habits re-occurring. In other words, replace the habits, find new ways to do and then enjoy experiencing our new poise and gracefulness in movement.

Getting the hang of it?

OK, back against the wall, legs bent. When you're ready, and after *inhibiting*, *projecting* and *controlling*, walk away slowly from the wall for a few steps. What does it feel like? And no, you don't have to walk around like this all the time. Just take a few steps in this new position. It's not right or wrong – it's just new. You haven't walked around like this for a while, maybe not even in this lifetime, but a few million years ago humans were walking like this all the time. It's the missing step between walking on all fours and walking upright.

As you walk around for a few steps let all the tension go. I bet you'll be holding your chest stiffly. Let your arms hang loosely and make the 'ahhh' sound we did earlier. Lighten up and let it all go.

Now walk backwards to the wall and see which bit touches first. I bet it was the buttocks. Walk away and walk backwards. Which bit now? Again the buttocks. And it will be for quite a while. When you do the standing against the wall in the mornings and evenings, walk away like this and see how quickly you revert to your old walk, and ask yourself why. There should be a nice in-between stage – in between this funny new walk and your funny old walk there is a stage of lightness and grace. As you pass through it see if you can feel it. By experiencing it a couple of times it will become familiar.

Are you sitting comfortably?

I want you to arrange three seating positions:

1 a standard hard-backed chair, like a kitchen chair
2 a couple of telephone directories on the floor to a height of about 15 cm (6 in) – or the distance between your fingertips and wrist
3 nothing at all.

I want you to sit first in the chair and notice where all the bits of you end up. How's your back? Your head? Your torso? Your legs and feet? These aren't trick questions – there's no right or wrong. Just have a look at yourself and see where you put everything.

Now sit cross-legged on the pile of directories. You can let your legs splay out in front of you with just your ankles crossed if it's more comfortable. Or you can raise your knees. Or splay your legs out completely. Again where is everything? How does it feel?

Now sit on the floor with nothing to support you. You can try to sit cross-legged or again splay your legs. How is everything this time?

Choosing our seating position

Now I want you to decide which of these three positions you would choose if you could choose only one to keep for the rest of your life. I don't know about you, but I'd go for the pile of directories. It's a nice height. There's plenty of choice about where I can put my legs. It feels comfortable and natural. I can't slump and, most importantly, I can sit there for hours without getting uncomfortable. So why is my desk at a regulation height, forcing me to sit on a hard chair? It's off to Japan for me where they understand these things. The second sitting position is close to our natural sitting position – the squat. Most people say they can't squat, but it's probably been a few years since they tried. You don't have to try squatting, but do think about your seating. Its height is now your choice, as it is mine. We have control and can make changes. But first we have to be aware that there might be a problem.

I'll extend your choice and throw in a comfortable, squishy old sofa. You now have four seating arrangements to choose from. Which would you go for? I do hope you were very keen and said 'the squatting position on the telephone directories'. Good, I'll have that old sofa if you don't want it. There are no right or wrong answers!

Emotional contortionists

Time to watch television. I want you to curl up on that old squishy sofa, while you've still got it, and watch some soaps. Good old-fashioned soaps. You can choose which, but not your favourites that you watch all the time. Choose new soaps. Have a pen and paper handy and I want you to watch carefully. Not for a good plot or good or bad acting. I want you to watch for emotions and feelings. You know the sort of thing – anger, worry, love, joy, depression, confusion. All the range of emotions we humans have to go through. Watch what the actors do to express those feelings with their bodies. Especially, watch their heads and shoulders.

After you've watched for a while, I want you to turn off the television and try to imitate what you've seen.

Now I want you to act out those emotions yourself – you can do this privately in the bathroom if you prefer. Don't speak, just let your body act out how *you* feel when you're angry or happy or worried or thoughtful. See what your body does each time.

For the next few days I want you to watch yourself very carefully. As each of these feelings occurs naturally be aware and see how close to the actual body movement you were when you were alone in the bathroom. Did you get it right? Close? Or way out? How did the actors do?

Monitoring our feelings

Keep doing this. As the feelings occur, monitor what you do with your body, and keep asking 'Why?' Now ask yourself what sparks off the feelings and whether they are valid. Did you get angry because the post was late? Were you anxious because someone promised to phone and didn't? Did you feel elated because you thought you'd won the lottery and then depressed because you realized you'd forgotten to buy a ticket?

All those feelings, all those body movements, what did any of them achieve? Did getting angry get the post to you any quicker? I think not. But it did increase your tension. What did you do with the tension afterwards?

Before we begin any body movement – and that includes being emotionally contorted – we can choose to remember to *inhibit*, *project* and *control*. That way we don't need to respond to stimuli unnecessarily. That way we don't build up tension. That way we don't need to hold on to tension because we don't get it in the first place. That way we don't get out of alignment.

You made me do it

Let's clear up another popular misconception about feelings. Controlling our feelings does not make us robots: it makes us adults.

We can choose what we feel and the degree to which we feel it. 'Ah,' I hear you say, 'but what if someone makes me angry?' That's the misconception. No one can *make* you angry. They can do things that you can then choose to get angry about, but it's your choice as to whether you have the feeling and then the degree to which you have it. But you'll say, 'What if something dreadful happens to someone I love – I'll feel sad.' Yes you will, but it's because you choose to and sadness would be the right expression of your grief, just as anger might be the right expression for some other emotion. This isn't about not having feelings – it's about realizing that we generate those feelings, that they are not visited upon us from some outside source. It's the stimulus that's outside and the feeling that's inside. The stimulus sparks off the feeling but we can choose not to respond to that stimulus, or to respond to a lesser degree, or be aware we have responded and then let go of the tension once we have done with it. If you got angry because the post was late and then went and killed the person who delivered it, that would be extreme, wouldn't it?

So where do you draw the line? How much anger is appropriate? Ask yourself that the next time you get angry, and also ask yourself what it achieves. This is about letting go of tension and not wasting energy.

What emotions are appropriate?

Suppose you come home and find someone has stolen everything you own. You'd certainly feel yourself do a perfect example of the startle pattern. And afterwards? What emotion or feeling would be appropriate? And to what degree? There are no *right* answers.

Exercise

Off to the bathroom with you again. I want you to stare at yourself in the mirror. Look closely at your eyes, while trying not to let them move, and tell me the answer to the following questions:

1 What is 1394 divided by 7?
2 What is the capital of Thailand?
3 What is the biggest ocean in the world?

I don't want the answers. I want to know what your eyes did while you were working out the answers.

Now look in the mirror again and watch your eyes – try not to let them move – and tell me the earliest memory you have. What did your eyes do?

Our eyes move when we think

If you refuse to allow your eyes to move, you may find it quite hard to work out the answers to anything. If your eyes did move they probably moved to the right and up while you worked out the answers to the first questions, and down and to the left while you told me about your childhood. This proves nothing except we move our eyes when we think. It's a neat party trick to play with friends.

The *primary control* is the head–neck relationship. The head is the primary control of the whole body, and the eyes are the primary control of the head. Our eyes are very important to our primary control, our primary control is very important to our movement, and our movement is important to our alignment. Where our eyes are directed can influence the position of our head, which governs the rest of the body. Misdirect the eyes and the whole lot goes to pot. Direct the eyes and the whole lot comes together like a dream.

Go for a walk

Exercise

This one's as easy as watching the television. I want you to go for a walk. You can go anywhere and for as long as you like. All I want you to do is come back and report where your eyes have been. Where did they look – not what at – what did they do? Try this next time you walk to the shops. Don't concentrate on where you think your eyes should be, just observe yourself and see where your eyes go. Do they look up a lot? Look down? Do they scan the horizon?

Most people walk with their eyes looking down at their feet. This leads the head to drop forwards, and the neck and back follow until we have the often seen position – modern human. That's how most of us end up: bent, stooped, doubled up – call it what you want, it's a human form that's not aligned properly.

There are two ways we can avoid this. If I simply told you to stop watching your feet, that would do little good. You might try for a while, but you actually need to learn a new way of walking.

Exercise

I want you to take another walk and this time I want you to imagine that you are a robot from an alien planet. Inside your head there is not a brain or a mind but the most sophisticated and advanced computer in the universe. The computer has sensors that detect visual stimuli on the front surface of its mechanism. This robot is capable of 'seeing' and storing the visual images for long enough that it can 'remember' and not look again. As you walk, you can scan the ground in front – about 3 m (10 ft) ahead of you. The computer will store all the information you need about surface texture, lumps and bumps, and unevenness. The computer will direct your feet and place them for you perfectly. I know this sounds silly but try it – all you have to do is trust.

You don't have to imagine that your head contains the most powerful computer in the universe. It does – your brain. Trust it. You don't have to bend over and peer at the ground when you walk. Try looking ahead and not at your feet. You'll find you can walk perfectly well, even better than before. We lose the art of trusting our natural instincts and instead try to control everything by conscious thought. Relax and let it work the way it was intended.

Walking with awareness

You can also try *walking with awareness*. Stroll and look without thought of what you have to do later, or what you're going to have for supper. Your walking will take no longer. In fact, you may even walk faster because you'll be walking more efficiently. Take time to notice what's happening all around you.

Why we walk the way we do

I bet if you got a piece of paper and a pen you could write down the names of all the members of your family and close friends and be able to describe in quite accurate detail things about the way they walk, what sort of stride they take, or the noise they make putting their feet down, or the speed of their walk. We recognize people at a distance by their walk long before we can make out their features. And we're just like them. We walk the same way all the time. We might speed up or slow down, but basically we walk in much the same way all the time. Now watch how a small child walks – he or she will walk a few steps, skip a few, jump a couple of times, run a bit, walk some more, hop on one leg for a while, turn around and walk backwards, hop again, skip and generally drive you mad. 'Walk properly!' 'Keep still!' 'Stop jigging about!' All instructions we've heard from our parents from time to time when we were small. We learn to control our natural urge to be constantly moving, constantly changing, and we learn to adopt a rigid and learnt habit or pattern of movement. We can try walking in different ways. How many different types of walk are there? You could take long strides, or short. A long stride with one leg and a short stride with the other. You could turn your feet in, or out, or one in and one out. You could take one fast step and one slow step. There are as many different ways of walking as there are people who walk. Why have we adopted only one? Try changing your walk. Try skipping or jumping.

Puppets

As we walk we can imagine the string attached to the top of our heads pulling us up, holding and supporting us. This is not a movement: it is an imagining, a reprogramming. Just the subtlest thought that will be buried deeply in your subconscious and which actually works – you'll walk more lightly.

Bouncing on your toes

Exercise

Go back to standing with your back to the wall. Let the three points of reference touch and keep your knees fairly straight. Now I want you to take just one step forwards and I want you to do it in slow motion. What happens? Did you lean slightly to one side as you lifted your leg to take that step? I bet you did. That's how most of us walk. We pick up each leg and throw it forwards and swivel our weight on to the forward leg while we pick up the back leg and throw that one forwards. A different way to try walking forwards, and one that is impossible to do in slow motion, is to take that first step by just letting yourself fall forwards.

The weight of your head will act as a sort of pivot. You should find that this action makes you go up on to your toes and then you'll be obliged to take that first step without leaning to one side. You'll be walking forwards as naturally as a small child does, falling into each new step.

Try walking around for a bit on tip-toe. Try bouncing on your toes as you walk. Try running by falling into the next step. Try standing in the narrowest doorway you can and take that first step. If you're doing it the new way you'll be fine, but if you're still doing it the old way you'll either touch the sides of the doorway, or you'll get stuck. If you can't find a narrow enough doorway, try putting two poles in the ground in the garden, about the same width as your shoulders plus a little bit on each side. You could even try this just standing up against a wall. You'll lean to the side you start off on, so have the wall on that side.

Semi-supine position

Exercise

For this exercise you will need a pen and paper and a friend. I want you to ask your friend if they will watch you carefully as you perform a simple action and record exactly how you do it: exactly where you put each limb, each bit of your body, as you do it. Afterwards, you can keep this as a record of how you once did something and then we'll look at another way of doing it. Now go and get your friend.

I want you to place some books on the floor and stand next to them ready to get down into the *semi-supine position*. You only need a couple of books. I'll explain later how you can work out exactly how many and to what height. At the moment just have a few to prop up your head. From the standing position I want you to get down into the semi-supine while your friend records how you do it. You might, for instance, sit down first and then fall backwards, or squat down and then roll over into the position. Then I want you to get up again while your friend records that also. Again, for example, you might sit up, then stand up, or even, as I once saw, be able to spring completely upright by arching your back. Now you can thank your friend nicely and dispense with their services.

OK, so you've got your record — and I've seen some bizarre ways of getting down and up, so whatever you've got don't worry about it, it's just the way you used to do it. Now, I'm going to suggest a new way for you to do it. It's neither better nor worse, it's just new, and it puts a lot less strain on your body.

I'll go through it in stages. Then you can look at Figure 6.2 carefully, and then give it a try.

Getting down into the semi-supine position the new way

* **Stage 1** – Put the books on the floor and stand facing them a body's length away and one pace to the side of them. Let your arms hang loosely by your side and look straight ahead.
* **Stage 2** – Bring one leg backwards until it is one stride behind.
* **Stage 3** – From this position drop down on to one knee.
* **Stage 4** – Lean forwards while still looking straight ahead and, using the arm that is opposite the knee that is still up, put that hand flat on the floor in front of you and to one side.
* **Stage 5** – Bring the other arm forwards and, as you do so, put the other knee flat on the floor until you are in the crawl position.
* **Stage 6** – Swing your bottom over towards the space in front of the book and let your body follow until you curl round into the semi-supine position with your knees bent.
* **Stage 7** – Check the books are in the right place, then adjust your arms so that they are in the right place with each hand either side on your lower stomach and the elbows on the floor. Make the 'ahhh' sound and relax.

banish back pain with Alexander Technique

Figure 6.2 *Getting down into the semi-supine position.*

Getting up from the semi-supine position in the new way

Basically it's the same as getting down into the semi-supine but in reverse, with one additional point that is very important. We talked earlier about our eyes leading the movement. Well, in getting up from the semi-supine it is important to let our eyes lead us. First, though, we have to make a simple choice – which side to get up. We can get up to the right or to the left. It doesn't matter which, although it's important not to get into using one side as a habit – keep changing. Once we've made the decision we can get up (see Figure 6.3).

* **Stage 1** – Turn your eyes to the side you've chosen and let your head follow. As your head turns let your body follow and roll on to your side.
* **Stage 2** – Keep rolling until you are back in the crawl position.
* **Stage 3** – From the crawl position let your eyes lead the movement. You're going up, so that's where your eyes should be. Sink back on to your heels and, as you do so, bring your arms to your side with your fingertips just touching the floor and go up on to one knee.
* **Stage 4** – From one knee, still looking up and forwards, you can bring the other knee up and fall into your first step and away you go. Put your fingertips at the back of your neck for the first few times to make sure you aren't tempted to use your arms to lever yourself up from your knees.

Practise these new ways in slow motion until they become second nature. Eventually, your movements will become fluid and graceful. It doesn't put any strain or tension on any part of your body. Try this over the next few days and see how you get on. Remember, it's not better or worse, it's just new and less damaging.

How many books?

You'll need your friend again. When you're lying in the semi-supine get him or her to check the height of your head. It should be parallel and level with your back, not at an angle up or down (see Figure 6.4).

Figure 6.3 *Getting up from the semi-supine position.*

Too high   Too low   Aligned

Figure 6.4 *How to adjust the books for the semi-supine.*

What are we doing in the semi-supine?

You now know how to get down and up and how many books you need – but do you know what you're supposed to be doing while you're there? OK, your feet need to be positioned so that they are flat on the floor, parallel and about 50 cm (20 in) apart. Your knees are bent and should be relaxed. If they have a tendency to fall outwards, move your feet slightly further apart. If they have a tendency to fall inwards, move your feet slightly closer together. Your hands should be relaxed and placed lightly one either side of your lower stomach. Your elbows should be touching the floor. *Imagine* your whole torso lengthening and widening. Imagine yourself as liquid, about to flow into a relaxed puddle. The semi-supine position lets gravity work for a while in your favour. For so long it has been pulling you downwards, now you can use it to repair some of the damage it has caused. Gravity will pull your shoulders down into a more aligned position and help your back spread openly and widely.

Now sit up and lie down again to allow your back to lengthen. You may need to reposition the books.

If you want to know what your pelvis is doing while you are in this position, try putting your legs down flat on the floor and then bring them up again. Feel how your pelvis swivels and tilts backwards. That's a better alignment for it and one it gets little chance to use with modern living.

Summary

So now you know how to get down, get up and lie there in between. Use this position twice a day for 15 minutes each time, or as long as you feel you can to begin with, and build up. If your knees get tired, you can put them down, but only one at a time and only for a few moments.

The semi-supine will correct misalignment, teach you a useful relaxation position and help your back to lengthen and widen.

In this chapter we have looked at:
* defining the Alexander Technique
* misconceptions about *inhibiting*, *conscious projecting* and *primary control*
* the best *use* of ourselves
* realigning ourselves
* how we get out of alignment
* choosing our seating position
* how our emotions can change our body shape
* a new way of walking
* the *semi-supine*.

Conclusions

* We need to be constantly adapting and changing.
* We need to be aware of how much we move by habit and, if those habits are not done according to the best principles of body design, change them.

Notes

<u>_Notes_</u>

Notes

Notes

Notes